Gluten-Free for Beginners
How to Be Gluten-Free and Healthy

Written By: James L. Shirley

A Gift For You!

We have a special gift for you! Visit http://HappyGlutenFree.com/Ingredient-Reference to get a FREE copy of our new Gluten-Free Ingredient Reference. You'll also get insightful information about the gluten-free diet delivered straight to your inbox.

Table of Contents

Introduction

What if you could wake up feeling great and have energy to last all day? And what if you didn't have to take any pills or supplements or join a gym or exercise regularly to get all that energy? What would you do? Imagine the possibilities! You could finally get out and do those things you've dreamed of doing!

For many, going on a gluten-free diet is the way to start feeling better right away. In this book I will show you how to be gluten-free by giving you a step-by-step process that really works.

Can you imagine living without unpleasant symptoms like stomach aches, headaches, or lethargy? Wouldn't it be wonderful if you could eat what you want and not worry about getting sick?

My name is James Shirley. I know what it's like to worry about what to eat. My family and I have been eating gluten-free for over five years. I especially know how hard it can be to sort through mountains of advice and medical jargon in search of simple answers for what to do next.

Back in 2007, my 18-month old daughter was diagnosed with celiac disease (my wife and I were relieved to finally know what was wrong, since so many horrible things had coursed through our minds). We decided to go 100% gluten-free to help our family live a healthier lifestyle. Even though my wife,

Karen, and I began reading everything we could find, we still had many unanswered questions.

While it was very difficult at first, day-by-day day we saw our daughter getting better. What could be more inspiring than that! So we continued taking notes, checking labels, and absorbing everything we could find. And over the years we became experts by trial and error.

In 2011, I took the list of gluten-free food my wife and I had compiled and turned it into a book called Gluten-Free Diet: A Shopping Guide. In 2013, the guide became a best seller and has a near five-star rating on Amazon.com.

Then in 2015, I took our actual experience of going gluten-free and turned it into this book you're reading right now: *Gluten-Free for Beginners*.

How does *Gluten-Free for Beginners* differ from all the other gluten-free guides?

During my research I found that most people interested in going on a gluten-free diet want practical advice in language that is easy to understand. So I eliminated medical or technical jargon (except where pertinent) to make this book as understandable as possible.

In *Gluten-Free for Beginners* you will learn how to successfully live a gluten-free life (information you can start using immediately). The lessons are delivered through ten simple concepts. And each concept has actionable information you can start using today.

From suggesting what to eat over the next week to what products you can buy at the supermarket, *Gluten-Free for Beginners* provides the framework you need to be gluten-free.

The book answers questions like:

- What is gluten?
- What are the symptoms of gluten intolerance and celiac disease?
- How do you begin a gluten-free diet?
- What is cross-contamination, and why does this matter?
- How do you make your kitchen gluten-free?
- How do you eat gluten-free outside your home?
- How do you spot gluten in a list of ingredients?
- What food can you eat?
- What food should you avoid?
- How do you manage the cost of gluten-free food?

Wouldn't it be nice to start feeling your best today? So let's get started as I know you'll enjoy what you're about to read!

Attention: Several people have proofread this book before it was released, but you may see errors we missed. If you find any and you're the first to report them, I'll send you a free gift! Send to:jim@happyglutenfree.com

Chapter 1: Knowing Gluten

This chapter will introduce you to important information you should know about gluten and being gluten-free. You'll want to know because once people find out you're gluten-free they will ask you to explain what gluten is and why it is an issue. In essence, YOU will become the expert!

What Is Gluten?

Let's start with a definition of gluten from Webster's Dictionary:

"A tenacious elastic protein substance especially of wheat flour that gives cohesiveness to dough."

The Concise Encyclopedia gives a more detailed explanation:

"Mixture of proteins not readily soluble in water that occurs in wheat and most other cereal grains. Its presence in flour makes production of leavened baked goods possible because the chainlike gluten molecules form an elastic network that traps carbon dioxide gas and expands with it. The properties of gluten vary with its composition, which differs according to the source. Thus, doughs range from soft and extensible to tough and elastic, depending on the gluten in the flours."

These definitions, however, leave out critical details about eating gluten-free.

As stated gluten is a protein in cereal grains, but it shows up in much more than just dough and wheat products. The common definition of gluten in the medical community (and as I refer to it throughout the book) is:

"A protein composite that comes primarily from wheat, barley, and rye."

This is a much broader definition, and specifies other grains to avoid when going on a gluten-free diet.

The gluten in wheat, barley and rye is used in many ways -- not just in baked goods.

Not all gluten is bad for those eating a gluten-free diet. In particular, corn and rice gluten don't have the same protein structure as gluten from wheat, barley, or rye. In fact, you'll find that many gluten-free products are made from rice and corn.

How is Gluten Used?

Gluten has beneficial characteristics that make it a useful ingredient in a variety of food and products. Gluten...

- Adds elasticity
- Is a filler
- Is a thickener
- Adds protein
- Is a flavor enhancer
- Is a binder

Given the expanse of benefits, you'll find gluten in all kinds of food you come in contact with every day!

A few examples of food containing gluten that might surprise you (since they are not baked from dough) are:

- Salad dressing
- Soup
- Seasonings/spice mixes
- Licorice

- Soy sauce

In addition to food, gluten can be present in cosmetics, shampoos, and flavored drinks. The list of foods that contain gluten is long. It seems like just about everything has gluten in it when you are first starting out on this diet!

But wait! Have hope! Many foods and products are made without gluten, and they are made by brands you know and trust (which I'll discuss in upcoming chapters).

Before I go into the world of gluten-free foods, I want to help you understand why gluten can be an issue for some people.

Why is Gluten a Problem?

Now you know what gluten is and how it can be used. Why is it such a problem?

Gluten causes negative reactions for people with celiac disease (an autoimmune disease), or for people sensitive to gluten proteins.

Why would gluten cause this reaction? It's an unanswered question in the medical community, and there are many theories as to why. But what is known is that reactions do occur, and the causes are not "in your head" as some doctors and health professionals used to think (and, sadly, often still do).

Gluten sensitivity is real, and it reveals itself in many ways. For some, the reaction to gluten occurs on their skin; for others as indigestion. Others might have celiac disease. Health problems differ depending on what kind of gluten sensitivity a person might have.

First, there is non-celiac gluten sensitivity – also known as gluten intolerance. Gluten intolerance is not an auto-immune disease like celiac, but the symptoms can be quite similar. With gluten intolerance, problems can be digestive or allergic reactions. The resulting symptoms range from diarrhea and gas to lethargy and fogginess. It can also cause rashes, headaches, nasal congestion and a variety of other negative reactions that clear up when gluten is removed from the diet or topical products.

Then, there is celiac disease. Celiac is an auto-immune disease caused by gluten sensitivity. With celiac disease, gluten is a problem because the body believes gluten is something it should fight and this results in an immune response.

What is Celiac Disease?

Celiac disease is the most common autoimmune disorder in the world, and affects adults and children. As many as 1 in 100 healthy adults have celiac disease, and even more are likely to have it if they experience the typical symptoms.

Gluten specifically causes damage to small villi (hair-like threads that absorb nutrients from food) in the upper part of the small intestine. When gluten comes into contact with villi, the body sees it as an invasion – like from a virus or poison. The body's immune system reacts and attacks the gluten and this attack causes damage to the villi. When villi flatten the body can no longer absorb nutrients from food. And without proper nutrients conditions can occur such as osteoporosis, infertility, malnutrition, iron deficient anemia, and sometimes cancer.

How do people get celiac disease? Celiac is most likely to occur in individuals with a certain genetic makeup. They may not be born with the disease, but possess the genes to contract it. However, there are cases of people being diagnosed with it even though they don't have the genetic predisposition.

In some individuals celiac and associated symptoms can appear rather suddenly. But others may have celiac for years with no recognizable or "silent" symptoms. An unknown trigger can set off the disease in the body without any warning, and it is not consistent from person to person.

Celiac is not a food allergy, nor is it the same as gluten intolerance. It is not a cold or virus. Unfortunately, once celiac becomes active a person can have the disease for life. But other forms of gluten sensitivities may disappear over time.

How do you know if you have celiac disease or sensitivity to gluten? One way to tell is to be tested for it. Another way to tell is to recognize if you are experiencing the typical symptoms. The symptoms are classified in the medical community as classical, atypical, and silent.

What Are Symptoms of Celiac Disease and Gluten Sensitivity?

Many possible symptoms exist for celiac disease and gluten sensitivity. And to make matters more complicated, each person has their own unique signs of it.

Should you be tested for celiac disease? If you, your children or anyone in your extended family have symptoms like those outlined below then yes, it's a good idea to talk to your doctor about getting tested.

It is important to have an official celiac diagnosis before going on a gluten-free diet. Once you switch to eating gluten-free, it becomes difficult for doctors to use the more standard tests to make a viable diagnosis.

Standardized tests detect how the body reacts to gluten both in blood work and how villi in the small intestine look. The moment you start eating gluten-free your body's -- if it's sensitive to gluten -- healing process begins, which makes getting an accurate diagnosis more difficult.

Classical symptoms differ between adults, young adults, and children. (Please keep in mind I'm not a physician. The lists below are an aggregation of information from books, the Internet, and my own personal experience.)

CHILD SYMPTOMS

- Diarrhea
- Stunted growth, or "failure to thrive" as some physicians call it
- Large, distended belly
- Child looks like they are starving or malnourished
- Vomiting after meals
- Decreased appetite
- Unable to gain weight, or are losing weight
- Irritability
- Fatigue
- Constipation

Although this isn't a complete list, these are the most common symptoms Infants and children with sensitivity to gluten tend to have digestive symptoms. If they are not getting the nutrition they need, it becomes obvious very quickly.

While listing these symptoms I became emotional thinking about our daughter when we were struggling to figure out what was wrong. After all these years it's still difficult to get doctors to order the tests for celiac disease, but this is slowly changing. If your doctor dismisses your concerns about gluten or is not knowledgeable about the disease, find one who is. If you see these symptoms in your child, be persistent and get the tests done! The sooner you know what is going on, the healthier your child's life will be.

ADULT SYMPTOMS

- Diarrhea
- Stunted growth
- Abdominal pain
- Bloated with gas
- Weight loss / underweight
- Fatigue
- Irritability
- Depression
- Persistent skin rash

SYMPTOMS FOR ADULTS

- Brain fog
- Osteoporosis
- Depression
- Joint pain
- Arthritis
- Chronic diarrhea

ATYPICAL AND SILENT SYMPTOMS

- Iron deficiency
- Anemia
- Gallbladder issues
- Persistent skin rash
- Dermatitis Herpetiformis
- Folic acid deficiency
- Unexplained infertility

It's common for adults to have multiple symptoms as well. Sometimes adults are asymptomatic until some other secondary disease like diabetes reveals they also have celiac.

If the symptoms above describe you, your child or a relative, it is important to see a doctor to determine if the problem is indeed celiac disease.

Thankfully, celiac and its symptoms are treatable by eating a gluten-free diet. Isn't it nice to know that simply changing your diet could be a cure? No surgery, no medicine … just smart, healthy eating.

How Are Celiac Disease and Gluten Intolerance Cured?

At the risk of stating the obvious, the way to be 100% gluten-free is to stop consuming gluten. Period!

The time it takes to get healthy and symptom-free varies from weeks to months, and can stretch to years for people who have lived a long time with undiagnosed celiac disease. Most celiac and gluten sensitive people start to feel better within days of beginning a gluten-free diet. Yes, it can happen that quickly!

Summary

- In this chapter you learned that gluten is a microscopic protein that comes from wheat, barley, and rye.
- You learned that the gluten protein can cause unpleasant reactions in people sensitive to it.
- Celiac disease is the most common autoimmune disorder in the world, and people who have it must eat a gluten-free diet for life.

- The symptoms for gluten sensitivity and celiac disease are varied and unique to each individual. Therefore, it is important to get tested for celiac disease if you experience any symptoms before you embark on a gluten-free diet.
- The way to treat gluten sensitivity and celiac disease is by going on a gluten-free diet.

But eating gluten-free is not easy. Or is it? Eating gluten-free can be made much easier if you have a good plan in place.

Chapter 2: Preparing to Eat Gluten-Free

The first few weeks on a gluten-free diet are the toughest. In particular, it is confusing to know what to eat and where to buy it. You may feel a sense of loss at the thought of the lifestyle change you're facing. But thorough planning and determination will help you get past the sense of loss.

In this chapter I will discuss a process you can use to be confidently gluten-free. I will show you how to track your progress, create a meal plan for a full week, and how to formulate a comprehensive grocery shopping list.

How to Track Your Progress

The amount of information relating to eating gluten-free is overwhelming. How can you possibly manage all the information? You can prevent being overwhelmed by keeping track of important information and your progress in a journal.

Bring your journal with you when you visit your doctor or nutritionist, as they may have tips you'll want to jot down. Reviewing it on a regular basis can show you what is going well, and where you need help as you transition to eating gluten-free.

Here are some ideas of things to note in your journal:

- Gluten-free foods you like
- Questions you have
- Meal ideas
- Date / time of moments you don't feel well and what you ate beforehand
- How you feel since being on a gluten-free diet

A three-ring binder with paper and folders makes a great journal. Use the folders to keep handouts, magazine clippings, Internet printouts and other information you collect. Use the paper to take notes and record details of how things are progressing.

If you find a recipe or product you love, make a note of it. When you make a mistake (and you will), make a note of that as well.

Keep track of symptoms. Note which food seems to work and those you should avoid (your body's responses will gives you clues). Logging successes and failures helps track your progress and accelerates the learning curve.

Organize your binder by sections such as Recipes, Notes, Products, and Medical. This will help you keep the information organized and ready to use. It's your personal journal, so make sure it fits your lifestyle.

You could also create and use an electronic journal. Programs like Evernote make note taking very easy. Plus with Evernote, you can capture pictures of recipes with your Smart phone, download pages from the Internet, and all the information can be organized into folders that can be shared between your computer, phone, and tablet.

Now that you have a solid plan for keeping track of how your gluten-free diet is going, it's time to plan for what to eat during your first week. (Even if you already eat gluten-free, it is helpful to go through the exercise of planning your meals in advance.)

How to Get Started

In this section you'll find meal and snack ideas for a full seven days, as well as tips for handling some common challenges.

During the first week you should focus on incorporating and cooking gluten-free food, as knowing what to eat each day can be a challenge.

This One Week Meal Plan includes suggestions for breakfast, lunch, and dinner (five of the seven breakfasts are great for busy workday mornings). These are all meals to cook at home. These are designed to be relatively simple to prepare until you get more comfortable with cooking gluten-free. (It's a given that all components should be gluten-free):

One Week Meal Plan

Recipes for these meals are located at the back of the book. Click the Table Of Contents and then choose "Recipes".

Breakfast
- Yogurt with fresh fruit
- General Mills Chex cereal (except Wheat Chex) and fruit – look on the front of the box for "gluten-free"
- Scrambled eggs and sausage
- Poached egg with sliced red pepper
- Bagel (Udi's is a widely available brand) with cream cheese
- Pancakes, scrambled eggs, fruit salad

- Breakfast tacos

Lunch
- Sandwich (gluten-free bread, Hormel Natural Selections packaged deli meat, sliced cheese)
- Corn tortilla quesadilla
- Chef salad
- Grilled cheese sandwich with tomato soup (Annie's is one example)
- Fruit and protein shake (i.e., Arbonne's protein mix)
- Nachos
- Baked potato with steamed vegetables

Dinner
- Tacos
- Burger and fries
- Salad
- Pasta with sauce
- Beef and broccoli stir fry
- Chicken enchiladas with corn tortillas
- Sweet and sour pork

Snacks
- Baby carrots
- Lay's Classic Potato Chips
- Cool Ranch Doritos
- Tootsie Rolls

- Peanut M&M's
- Crunchmaster Multi-Grain Crackers
- Betty Crocker Fruit Roll-Ups
- Musselman's Cinnamon Apple Sauce
- Frito Lay Cashews

This is a total of 21 meals to use over seven days, so you can mix and match to create meals for each day.

The next step is to make a grocery list from your meal planning.

How to Make a Grocery List

Although the trend for providing gluten-free products to consumers is on the rise, finding appealing food can be challenging. To make the search easier you should have a grocery list to take with you to the supermarket.

Research gluten-free alternatives for each item on your list in case the supermarket is out of the product you're looking for, and write them next to the item. For example, the start of a grocery list for the One Week Meal Plan could look like the one below (in the chapter titled "Be Confident" I suggest many more gluten-free options):

Produce
- Head of lettuce
- Mixed greens
- Tomato

- Garlic
- Onion
- Bell peppers
- Potatoes
- Fresh fruit (whatever is in season that you like)

Meat
- Ground beef
- Pork chops
- Chicken breasts
- Beef for stir fry
- Lunch meat (Hormel Natural Selections, Oscar Mayer)

Dairy
- Cheddar cheese
- Monterey Jack cheese (Kraft or Tillamook)
- Eggs
- Sour cream (Frigo, Tillamook)
- Yogurt (Stonyfield, Yoplait if labeled gluten-free)

Miscellaneous
- Cereal (General Mills Chex– cinnamon, chocolate, honey nut, rice, corn)
- Taco shells (Ortega)
- Corn tortillas (Mission, Ortega)
- Tortilla chips (On the Border, Tostitos)
- Pasta (Tinkyada, DeBoles)

Depending on where you live, it could be hard to find gluten-free products. But that shouldn't limit you as you can order the food online and have it shipped to your door. These websites sell gluten-free products at competitive prices:

Amazon.com: In addition, you get free two-day shipping and cheap overnight shipping with an Amazon Prime membership.

Celiac.com - The Gluten-Free Mall: Is one of the original online gluten-free supermarkets.

Summary

- Keep a journal where you can note questions, important tips, gluten-free food, and organize printouts, recipes and research material.
- Plan your meals to help make it easier to shop and eat gluten-free.
- Make a grocery list with gluten-free brands so you know exactly what to buy.

Maintaining a gluten-free diet can seem daunting when you think of it in terms of weeks or months, so take it one day at a time. Baby steps... baby steps... baby steps!

If you accidentally eat food containing gluten, address your physical symptoms, work on feeling better, and don't beat yourself up about it. Being on a gluten-free diet will become second nature and an inherent part of your healthier lifestyle.

Chapter 3: Be Aware of Cross Contamination

Sometimes all it takes is a couple crumbs of the wrong food to make you feel ill. Since something that small can cause problems, you have to avoid cross-contaminating your food with gluten.

Cross-contamination is when gluten-free food is anywhere near food that contains gluten. It can occur in many different places including restaurants, jars of condiments, and even on your own kitchen counter.

But how can you make sure your gluten-free food is safe from cross-contamination? You'll need to take steps to understand what cross-contamination is; know how and where it happens; and know how to be safe.

What is Cross-Contamination?

Cross-contamination -- as it's referred to here -- is when you get something containing gluten (like bread crumbs) mixed in with your gluten-free food. Or it can happen when gluten-free food is cooked with the same appliance or in cookware as food containing gluten.

Gluten, even though microscopic, is a living organism. Most celiac and gluten intolerant individuals have to ingest it to get a reaction. Some are sensitive enough that just breathing flour dust or using topical products, such as shampoo or lotion, that contain gluten can cause a negative reaction. Even crumbs from a crouton can cause gluten sensitive individuals to have a reaction after eating a salad.

You can avoid ingesting unwanted gluten by being aware of the different places where cross-contamination can occur. For example, a deep fryer is pretty obvious as people tend to fry different food in the same oil. But where else can your otherwise gluten-free food be cross-contaminated?

Where Can Cross-Contamination Occur?

Cross-contamination can occur in your home, at your friend's home, or at a restaurant. Anywhere that food is served and eaten.

It happens most often on kitchen countertops, grills or griddles. Or it can occur when bread crumbs are transferred from utensils to things like butter, mayonnaise or a jelly jar.

Cross-contamination happens when wheat flour dust is left on the same cutting board where vegetables have been sliced.

A pasta strainer is another problem area. Even if your gluten-free pasta is cooked separately, the pasta might be put in a contaminated container (and washing it with cold water won't get rid of all the cross-contamination).

Maybe you're looking forward to a summertime barbecue. Chicken or burgers cooked on the same grill where buns are toasted can cause you to get sick if you're gluten sensitive. And don't forget that restaurants use grills to cook all sorts of food, so cross-contamination can certainly occur there.

A salad mixed with croutons is contaminated even if you remove all the croutons.

Unfortunately, there are numerous ways your gluten-free meal could accidentally get gluten in it and make you ill. But you still have to eat and go on with your life, so how can you make sure your food is safe?

How Can You Be Sure Your Food is Safe At Home?

Your kitchen is an area you can control. Since you can make the decision where to store, clean and cook food, it should be a reliably safe place to make gluten-free meals. Here are some ways to protect food from cross-contamination:

- Make sure cooking surfaces are clean, and that no crumbs, flour dust, or other potentially harmful by-products are left on countertops.
- Make sure pots, pans, and cooking utensils are scrubbed clean.
- Use dedicated gluten-free cutting boards and pasta strainers. Never use them for anything else.
- Keep your food safe by boldly labeling the containers.
- Keep your gluten-free food sealed and separate from gluten food.
- Make sure everyone in your household knows how to handle the food, cookware, and post-cooking cleanup, even if they don't have gluten issues. Their lack of diligence can cause other family members to become ill.

These are the main points to consider in your kitchen (I'll talk about how to set up the kitchen to be gluten-free later on).

How Can You Be Sure Your Food is Safe Away From Home?

It is more challenging to prevent cross-contamination outside of your home. It is impossible to see what's going on in the restaurant's kitchen. You know someone is preparing your food, but you can't see how it's being prepared. For instance, it's most likely that fries are cooked in the same fryer as other food, so I almost always avoid them or anything that might be cooked in a fryer as it's not worth the risk.

So how *can* you protect yourself from cross-contamination when you can't see the kitchen or the people handling your food? You can ask the wait staff questions about how the food is prepared. Don't hesitate to ask. It's the restaurant's responsibility to provide safe eating for its clientele, and you're paying for the meal!

Ask questions from different angles, such as:

You:
- *Are your fries gluten-free?*
- *Are the fries cooked in the same fryer as other food?*

- *How can I be guaranteed my food hasn't been contaminated with food containing gluten?*
- *What procedures does your restaurant use to keep your food gluten-free?*
- *How do you prevent food from getting cross-contaminated with gluten in your kitchen?*
- *I ask these questions because I'm very sensitive to gluten, and you don't want me getting sick at the dinner table.*

Waiter:

I'll go ask the chef.

See how you can get clarification by asking follow-up questions? Of course there are no guarantees, but the willingness of the wait staff and chef to answer them shows good intent.

It's okay to ask these same kinds of questions of friends and family too. They wouldn't want to cook something that makes you feel bad! Don't hesitate to ask to read the labels of the ingredients they used, where they bought the food (i.e., organic store or standard supermarket), and how they cooked it.

Just make sure they know how much it means to have someone willing to make you a meal that won't make you ill, and that they should not take your tummy issues personally. With the rising awareness of celiac disease and gluten issues, many people are well aware of the problems it can cause.

Summary

- All it takes is a crumb or two to cross-contaminate a gluten-free meal.
- Contamination can happen in restaurants and even in your own kitchen.
- You can protect food prepared in your kitchen by making sure cooking surfaces are sanitized, and your cookware is dedicated gluten-free. Also, be sure all gluten-free food containers or packages are clearly labeled to prevent accidental use.
- You can protect yourself by asking questions about how your food is prepared outside the home.

Unfortunately, you'll occasionally get gluten in a meal, as there's no way to avoid it 100% of the time. Be thankful to everyone who tries to accommodate you even if they sometimes fail. Your graciousness will encourage them to keep trying for you and for others they'll be cooking for! Be diligent about asking questions to clarify how your food was prepared, and don't be afraid to pass if something doesn't sound right.

A mantra to live by is "If you don't know, don't eat it!"

The one place you should be able to avoid getting gluten cross-contamination is in your kitchen. But how can you make sure it's always a safe place to eat and prepare gluten-free meals? I'll cover that in the next chapter.

Chapter 4: GF At Home

Your kitchen is the one place where you should be able to safely prepare and eat gluten-free meals. But how can you make that happen? By following a step-by-step process, you and your family can live and cook in a gluten-free zone free from cross-contamination.

Before you convert your pantry and refrigerator to accommodate gluten-free groceries, you'll need a well-constructed plan. The first question to ask should be whether or not the kitchen can become 100% dedicated gluten-free, which will be determined by how many family members are switching to the new diet plan.

Many people across the country are doing the same thing, so you won't be alone in your decision. Karen and I know of households where only one or two members are no longer eating gluten and have made their kitchens very safe.

Have You Already Kicked Gluten Out of Your House?

As I previously mentioned, when my daughter was diagnosed with celiac disease my wife and I decided our family would become gluten-free. Switching was difficult at times, but watching her grow into a healthy young girl has been worth all the effort.

Once you transition to a gluten-free diet you won't have to worry about cross-contamination, labeling, or storing food in special bins. But you have to make sure your home truly is free of gluten.

If you have already turned your house gluten-free, it is still worth skimming the rest of this chapter to make sure you have everything covered. And occasionally, you end up cooking in a kitchen that is not yours – like when you are on vacation. Reading through this information will help you be prepared for those situations.

How to Protect Food in a Shared Kitchen

Although it's possible to share gluten-free with non-gluten items, you'll need to take extra precautions to make sure your gluten-free food stays safe. Find designated shelf space in the pantry and fridge that you can use for non-gluten items.

Pantry

Keeping gluten-free items in sealed containers helps in a couple of ways. First, it ensures your gluten-free food won't become contaminated by any sneaky food particles. And second, the container is portable so it's easy to transport food from place to place.

When the dedicated space is ready to go, you can stock your shelves with items like gluten-free cereals, crackers, and flour. Then label them on all sides as such with a permanent marker, or big, legible labels so there's no question about what's in the container.

Kitchen

In some cases, you will have both gluten and non-gluten items. Using a utensil (i.e., spreading a condiment on a sandwich with a knife) exposed to food containing gluten risks causing cross-contamination. So it's safer to have two sets of more commonly used items in a shared kitchen. For example, plan to have two of things like mustard, butter, jam and peanut butter -- making sure to label the correct ones as gluten-free.

Salad dressing, condiments, and perishable food can be stored on the shelves you've chosen to be gluten-free. It is a good idea to put a big label on the shelves stating "Gluten-Free" so that others in the household know to leave the food alone.

If you have a shared kitchen you should also have dedicated cookware (i.e. a pasta strainer, cutting board, cookie sheets, pots and pans, etc.). Keep them on the designated shelf in the pantry.

If several people cook in the kitchen an idea is to buy brightly colored utensils and cookware. Or use bright labels. Then everyone in your house knows that all the cookware with red on it is your gluten-free cookware. It's just one more way to help prevent accidental cross-contamination.

Now that you have an idea of how to make your kitchen safely gluten-free, it's time to finish your plan and share it with your household.

Sharing Your Plan

Have you already thought of ways to make room for gluten-free food in your kitchen? If you share your kitchen with others it is a good idea to think out your gluten-free kitchen strategy first and share it with the people you live with.

By making a plan and sharing it with everyone in your house, you will be educating them on your strategy. When those you live with know your plan, they will be less likely to accidentally cause cross contamination or eat your expensive cookies.

Write a simple but comprehensive outline in your journal using topics such as:

- How foods will be labeled and stored.
- Where the food will be stored.

- Where you will keep gluten-free cookware, appliances and utensils.
- How you plan to prepare the meals.

Anything else specific to your situation can be added as you become more familiar with your new lifestyle.

Once your plan is complete, convene a meeting with all members of your household. Discuss the steps in detail, and be open to receiving feedback as you might get some good suggestions. Going gluten-free can seem daunting at first.

By the way, I talk mostly about family because that's the lifestyle I have. But this guide also works for roommates and guests – anyone who will be eating in your home who needs to know about your situation.

Now you're ready to put your plan into action, but where do you begin? Next I'll give you checklists to help you get your kitchen safely gluten-free.

Checklist for Shared Kitchens

If you are sharing your kitchen with gluten food (and presumably the people who eat that food) then follow this list to make sure you have a safe place to prepare and eat your meals. The recommendations for finding space in your kitchen are pretty conservative. If you have room in your kitchen, claim as much space as you can!

Pick a shelf or drawer in the refrigerator that will be yours. Find a new spot for the foods that are there now. Get a towel and thoroughly clean the shelf or drawer. Now label this space gluten-free.

- Pick a shelf in the pantry or cupboard that will be yours. Find a new home for the stuff presently in that space. Clean it well. Now label this space gluten-free.

- Clean out your utensil holder and plan to start doing this on a regular basis if the utensil drawer is near a place where others prepare food with gluten in it.

- Clean out your cooking utensils drawer (if you have one) and plan to clean it out periodically if it attracts crumbs.

- Pick out a food storage container set that you can use for leftovers.

- Buy a couple of cooking utensils like spoons and spatulas

- It is not mandatory to buy a separate muffin pan, cookie sheet, or cutting board, but it is the safest way to go if you can afford it. If you plan to share these items with gluten foods, make sure they are extra super clean before you use them for gluten-free cooking.

- Get a toaster or toaster oven eventually. You can get by with sharing a toaster with everyone else if you buy some Toastabags – which are Teflon envelopes that protect your bread or bagel from touching any crumbs in the toaster. They are inexpensive to buy on Amazon.com.

- Start buying gluten-free foods!

Checklist for Making Your Kitchen Dedicated Gluten-Free

If you live alone or everyone you live with is going gluten-free, I recommend following these steps to make your kitchen safe from cross-contamination.

1. Eliminate all food containing wheat, barley, rye, or oats as an ingredient.

2. Eliminate any food items that might be cross-contaminated. For example, condiments (like ketchup, mustard and mayonnaise), spreads (like peanut butter), and jars of jam might be contaminated with gluten crumbs.

3. Give away plastic food storage containers that have held gluten food.

4. Give away strainers, the toaster, and any utensils and cookware that might be contaminated (but hold on to your toaster oven if you have one because you can clean it out and cook your foods on aluminum foil)

5. Clean, clean, clean! Sanitize the utensil drawer, and scrub pots and pans and baking sheets. Sanitize the refrigerator,

pantry, and cupboards to make sure there are no loose crumbs floating around. Scrub cutting boards – especially plastic and wood ones because their surfaces are absorbent and can contain residue from earlier use. White vinegar and water works great as you're not using toxic chemicals, and it smells so clean. Also after you've cleaned the refrigerator, it wouldn't hurt to wash the walls with water and baking soda as it organically deodorizes and sanitizes.

Now you can start fresh with new utensils, cookie sheets, a new toaster, new food storage containers, and a new strainer -- one of everything will suffice. And if buying new isn't possible on your budget, you can get by with sanitizing existing cookie sheets, utensils, and storage containers really, really well. However, the toaster still has to go, as there's no way to get it 100% gluten-free from prior use.

Then start filling your cabinets with gluten-free food, and you're on your way!

Summary

- Decide whether you'll have both gluten and non-gluten food in the kitchen or if you can make your kitchen completely gluten-free.
- If you have to share your kitchen with both gluten and non-gluten (depending on who

will be using the new meal plan), share your plans with the entire household.
- Make sure the food, cookware, pantry, refrigerator and eating space are free of gluten.
- Thoroughly sanitize the kitchen, including the pantry and refrigerator.
- Designate clearly labeled storage spaces and containers as gluten-free to prevent cross-contamination.

Taking these precautions to make sure the food you eat and cookware you use are safe from gluten cross-contamination will give your body a chance to heal completely. Best of all you will start to feel so good you'll wonder why you didn't do this sooner!

Chapter 5: How to Eat Gluten-Free at Parties

Does your heart sink when someone invites you to a party? It would be nice to see everyone. But all that gluten! What can you safely eat or drink? Suddenly the party doesn't seem so appealing and you think of turning down the invitation.

Don't despair! With a little planning and preparation you can enjoy the party without worrying about accidentally eating gluten. Just because you're adapting to a new gluten-free lifestyle doesn't mean you need to give up being social and having fun!

How to Prepare for the Event

You should go the party, and you should be able to eat and drink like everyone else. But to enjoy yourself without obsessing about every little thing on a platter, you'll need to do some sleuthing beforehand.

Find out as much as you can about the food and beverages that will be served. Will there be vegetable and cheese trays? Will you be drinking soda and juice, or just cocktails? Would the host or hostess mind if you bring your own food and beverage?

The invitation might tell what they're serving, or you might know from having been to their house before. But if you don't know, don't hesitate to call and explain your situation. You might feel a bit embarrassed, but for the safety of your health you really need to know more information.

If the party is small and intimate, talk to the host about what's being served. If it's held at a hotel or restaurant, or is being professionally catered, then call ahead of time and ask if they offer any gluten-free options. You might be pleasantly surprised to find they have gluten-free food on the menu, or how easily certain items can be modified to your specifications.

Now that you've done your detective work, you'll need to figure out what to bring to the party.

What to Bring

Don't assume there will be gluten-free options when dining outside your home. Be prepared to bring your own gluten-free food and beverages. My wife and I always keep a stash of non-perishable items in our cars (she even has some in her purse), and I recommend you do the same as it allows you more flexibility to join last-minute activities.

If you've followed the suggestions above you know what sort of food will be served. So the next step is to either buy or prepare food that fits your needs such as vegetables, fruit, cheese, and gluten-free crackers (or a main dish if it's a sit-down dinner). If they do provide gluten-free options, you can bring a substitute if it doesn't appeal to you.

You may already have something in mind from your kitchen (i.e. gluten-free crackers and a vegetable dip). Many dressings, corn chips and salsas are gluten-free, but you can bring your own to be safe.

Dessert is often served at parties, and you should have the opportunity to indulge in something sweet too! Gluten-free cupcakes, brownies, and cookies are great options. You can bake something fresh to bring, or buy something on the way to the party.

To recap, you can't go wrong bringing gluten-free food such as:
- Chips
- Dip
- Crackers
- Dressing
- Salsa
- Cupcakes

- Brownies
- Cookies
- Cheese
- Vegetable tray
- Salad
- Fruit salad

You won't want to set your food next to something that could potentially contaminate yours, so don't forget to label the containers with your name and "gluten-free."

Now you know what to bring to the party. But what should you do when you show up with your own food?

What to Do When You Arrive

You show up ready to have a good time but what about all that food you brought? What should you do next?

First, say hello to the hosts and guests, and then head immediately to the kitchen.

If there's room, store your food in the refrigerator or on a counter safely away from other food. If not, then get a plate and serve yourself first. You don't have to eat it right away – you can set it aside somewhere out of the way. But if you're food will be blended in with all the other trays of food then there is potential for accidental cross-contamination. You don't want to get gluten after going to all that trouble to bring something safe! Keep everything low-key and don't make a big deal out of it. Your health is your main priority.

If you are at a dinner party where there are gluten-free options, find the catering manager or the host and let them know you are one of the people who needs a special meal. They will likely have some additional information for you. Plus, they can answer any questions you have.

Finally, keep your eyes and ears open. You might find someone else at the party with special dietary needs – even if it isn't gluten sensitivity or celiac disease. You could ask what sort of menu they're following and how they handle their dietary restrictions. Any education is good education!

But hold on a minute. You have the gluten-free food figured out, but what can you drink?

What to Drink

Now that you're settled in and are having a great time, you'll probably want something to drink. Fortunately, many beverages are gluten-free.

You know water is safe (preferably bottled and not tap), but you have to watch out for tea. Did you know that barley is an ingredient in some brands? I didn't either -- I just assumed it was, well, tea. Unless you know what the ingredient label says, avoid it. By the way, coffee is fine.

Many sodas such as Coke, Pepsi and their diet versions are safe. Juice is safe as long as it is 100% juice. Capri Sun is safe for kids if they are at the party as well.

Wine is safe as are tonic and soda water. Many experts in the gluten-free community agree that alcohol products like vodka, whiskey, gin, and tequila are safe because the distillation process removes all gluten.

But avoid beer as it can contain hops, malt, barley and/or wheat grain. However, there are several good gluten-free ones on the market, so if beer is your drink of choice you could make some calls ahead to liquor stores to see what they carry. BYOB is totally acceptable at many parties and barbecues.

Relax and enjoy yourself. Eat, drink and be merry now that you know you can have fun without worrying about getting sick!

Summary

The key to having fun at a party while remaining gluten-free is being prepared ahead of time. Find out as much information as you can about what food and beverages will be served.

- Bring your own gluten-free pre-labeled food and beverages! Even a simple plate of crackers and cheese can make you feel physically more comfortable and less conspicuous.
- When you first arrive, find a safe place to keep your food. If the refrigerator is too crowded, serve yourself immediately to prevent cross-contamination.
- Many beverages are gluten-free, including sodas like Coke and Pepsi, wine, vodka and whiskey. Juice is also a great option.

You can be gluten-free and still enjoy food at parties. Make the effort to come prepared with gluten-free food and snack options. With every party and event you attend, you'll become more educated about the right things to bring or to order beforehand.

Expectations from social events are different than eating at restaurants ... or are they? Eating out or at a party can produce similar obstacles, which is what I'll discuss in the next chapter.

Chapter 6: Eating Gluten-Free at Restaurants

Dining at restaurants gives you a chance to get out of your house and enjoy good food and your community. And it's great because you have no cooking or dishes to do.

But is it possible to eat out and eat gluten-free?

Is it Safe to Eat at Restaurants?

Yes, it can be safe to eat at restaurants. But certain risks come with dining out.

A restaurant kitchen is a beehive of activity. Multiple dishes are being prepared at the same time. Chefs and staff are busy preparing meals on shared work spaces, and food is often cooked in shared pots and pans (which is where the risk of cross-contamination comes into play). In all that chaos bread crumbs may accidentally fall into a salad container. So what you thought was going to be a tasty gluten-free salad causes you to feel ill.

Different people will be handling your food. The wait person takes your order, but a chef prepares the meal. Then someone else might bring the plate to your table. All of this switching around can increase the risk that something can become cross-contaminated.

Despite the risks, thousands of people sensitive to gluten dine out all the time and you can too. All you need is a few restaurants that offer a gluten-free menu, the answers to a few good questions, and the willpower to trust your instincts if something does not seem right.

How to Find Restaurants with Gluten-Free Food

Thanks to the Internet and smart phones, finding gluten-free restaurants is easier. And since going gluten-free has exploded in popularity, restaurants and people are aware of it more than ever.

With a little research you can find restaurants that have a gluten-free menu. If you're using the Internet, type in a search phrase like "gluten-free restaurant your hometown" which will give you available options.

If you have a Smart phone, there's an app called "Find Me Gluten-free" that uses your geographic location to find nearby restaurants.

Referrals can help find gems, so you can ask trusted people to suggest gluten-free restaurants. Or ask a favorite wait person at your local hang-out for menu recommendations.

Many restaurants don't want to lose customers, so they might work with you to accommodate your needs. But don't assume a restaurant will have gluten-free food, so do your due diligence ahead of time to find out if they do. It's best to know before you show up hungry and find there's nothing on the menu you can eat.

As of this writing, these particular restaurants offer gluten-free menus:

- Applebee's
- Bonefish Grill
- Boston Market
- California Pizza Kitchen

- Carrabba's Italian Grill
- Chick-fil-A
- Chipotle Mexican Grill
- In-N-Out Burger
- Le Peep Restaurants
- Noodles & Company
- Olive Garden
- On the Border
- Outback Steakhouse
- P.F. Chang's China Bistro
- Pei Wei Asian Diner
- Red Robin
- Uno Chicago Grill

Now that you know what to expect and have a few restaurant options, you're good, right? Wrong. It's still possible to get gluten if you're not careful. When you arrive at a restaurant it's important to immediately establish your dietary restrictions with the wait staff.

What to do When You Get to the Restaurant

Some wait staff know what it means to serve a meal gluten-free, some are eager to learn, some are empathetic, and some just don't care. So you may need to "educate" your server to make sure you get everything the way you want.

Rather than leaving all the research to your server, call the restaurant ahead of time. The hostess may or may not know the answers, but they can connect you with the manager or assistant manager (which would be ideal because they and the chefs know the menu and the kitchen well). Call during off-peak hours; otherwise, they may not have enough time to discuss your needs.

Below are some good questions to ask (feel free to add any particular questions relating to your special needs):

- What gluten-free menu items do they have?
- What precautions do they take to keep food gluten-free?
- If they serve pancakes or hamburgers, are the gluten-free ones cooked on the same griddle as the non-gluten?
- Is the salad pre-mixed with croutons or other gluten-containing toppings?
- Ask if you can be seated with a gluten-knowledgeable member of the wait staff as some servers are more aware than others.

Keep in mind that researching which restaurants serve gluten-free food only needs to be done periodically. It's a good idea to check every six months or so to see what changes have occurred -- and any time there is a change in management -- to ensure the same protocols for gluten-free dining are being followed.

But even if you know the restaurant has a gluten-free menu, you should talk with your server upon arrival to make sure they handle your order properly.

Always communicate to your wait person that you have to eat gluten-free. This is an outline of steps to follow when you arrive:

- Ask for the gluten-free menu before being seated.
- When your server comes to take your drink order, let them know you intend to order from the gluten-free menu.
- Ask if they can recommend any gluten-free appetizers. This is a great way to alert them that you'll be eating gluten-free throughout the meal.
- Ask which salad dressings are gluten-free (don't be surprised if they don't know as this usually isn't a topic of discussion in the kitchen). Places like Amazon.com sells gluten-free salad dressings in portable packets. It's a good idea to keep some in your car or handbag in case a restaurant can't tell you if its dressings are gluten-free.
- Confirm that your salad isn't pre-mixed with croutons or any toppings containing gluten.

Your meal should go well if the answers to all your questions have been answered to your satisfaction.

Another important point: When you plan to dine with a group, take charge for choosing where to go. That way, you'll be guaranteed to have gluten-free options!

Lastly, if your instincts tell you that something is not right, don't eat and don't be afraid to leave.

But what if you're asked to join the CEO of your company for dinner at the last minute? And what if the restaurant doesn't have a gluten-free menu? I'll talk about how to deal with that next.

How to Improvise

On occasion you'll end up in a situation where you need to dine at a restaurant that doesn't have a gluten-free menu. For instance, if you're traveling for work and you're asked to join your boss or colleague for dinner.

What should you do? You have options available. Of course, the obvious one is to decline (unless it means you'll upset your boss). Or you could join but not eat.

The other option is to improvise. Mention your needs to your server immediately upon arrival. Then look at the menu and see if you can find what should be a gluten-free item. Foods like grilled chicken or a side of vegetables can often be prepared safely for you by cooking them in a separate pan.

If the setting isn't conducive for discussing your dietary restrictions in front of your boss (as it would be embarrassing), excuse yourself to talk with the hostess. Or pull the server aside and let them know your special dietary restrictions.

If you're comfortable with the people at your table, tell the server you're allergic to gluten and you need to know what options they have. If they're not sure, suggest they send a manager or chef to see you and ask them what they recommend.

Or tell them what you prefer, such as grilled chicken along with steamed vegetables – all prepared on separate cookware. Meat is safe as long as it's cooked on a gluten-free surface and is unseasoned. You can also safely eat fruit, or a selection of vegetables.

Or you can order a salad with instructions like:

"I'd like a salad. Does that come with croutons or bread sticks? I need a salad that hasn't touched any bread whatsoever."

Ask for olive oil and a splash of lemon juice for dressing, a specialty vinaigrette (flavored vinegar and oil), or use one of those handy portable salad dressing packets I mentioned earlier.

You can usually find something safe to eat. It takes a little work and may not be exactly what you want, but it's only one meal and at least you won't go away hungry.

Summary

- It's generally safe to eat at restaurants that offer a gluten-free menu.

- You can find restaurants that offer a gluten-free menu by searching on the Internet, or using an app on your Smart phone.
- When you find a restaurant with a gluten-free menu, call ahead of time to discuss available options.
- When you first arrive at a restaurant, make sure the server knows you need to eat gluten-free. Ask questions to make sure they understand your needs. If they seemed confused or don't know what gluten-free is, talk to the manager or chef.
- If you're at a restaurant that doesn't offer a gluten-free menu, you can improvise by eating plain salad, fruit or vegetables. Don't forget to ask questions about toppings, bread sticks, etc.
- Dining out gives you the opportunity to get out of the house and enjoy food and community, and it provides a respite from cooking and cleaning dishes.

Yes, it can be riskier to eat at restaurants than at home. But most of the risks can be identified and minimized by asking questions. It wouldn't hurt to always have a list of questions handy so you don't forget something important. So I have taken the questions to ask restaurants and wait staff and put them on a separate page you can easily get to from the table of contents in this book. Simply go to the chapter titled "Restaurant Questions" at the end of this book.

Chapter 7: Vacationing Gluten-Free

Have you been to the Grand Canyon? Have you seen the Eiffel Tower? Do you dream of relaxing on the beach with a cool cocktail in your hand?

Will you be able to travel and see all you want to see and be gluten-free?

Actually, your dreams of travel can still come true. It just takes some planning and the willingness to be an explorer.

How to Plan a Successful Gluten-Free Vacation

A vacation is supposed to be relaxing, so you don't want to spend precious time stressing over what to eat and where. Making trips to the supermarket and eating on your bed while watching TV in a hotel room is NOT a vacation, nor is it relaxing. I know from experience, and you can learn from my mistakes.

Yes, you will be able to travel and eat gluten-free. But you'll need to follow a plan to make the most of your time away from home.

But What Will You Eat?

Now that you're eating gluten-free, going on a vacation requires researching what you have or don't have available at your destination.

These are the most important things to look for while doing your research:

- Where will you buy gluten-free food? Are there supermarkets or specialty stores nearby?
- What restaurants serve gluten-free food?
- Where can you stay that has a kitchen (or at least a refrigerator and stove)?

Sometimes your research will go well and you can comfortably book your vacation. But sometimes, research reveals that your vacation might be more difficult than anticipated. Maybe you can't find an affordable place to stay that meets your requirements. Or you can't find one single restaurant that serves gluten-free food. For one reason or another, things aren't falling into place like you hoped.

If possible, find an alternate vacation destination (I've experienced that a few times when planning a family trip). It's not easy – particularly if there is a specific place you want to go. However, I have a long list of places I would like to see and when one place doesn't seem like a fit, I just start researching the next place.

But how can you tell if a destination is good for gluten-free? I'll show you each of the steps I take when planning a trip.

How to Find Places to Buy Gluten-Free Food

Open an Internet browser and search for supermarkets in whatever destination you want to travel to, and be as specific as possible. Maybe you want to go to San Diego, California, so enter "San Diego supermarkets" in the search bar. If you want to stay on Coronado Island, be more specific by typing in "Supermarkets Coronado Island."

Note the location, phone number, and name of grocery stores that pop up. Call to see what gluten-free food they have. Check their website (if they have one) for any recognizable gluten-free items on their menu. A digital version of a circular in the local newspaper might show the food they carry.

Every supermarket has produce, meat, dairy and beverages, so you won't have to worry about food if you're not planning on eating in restaurants. But it would be nice to know if they have gluten-free items like cookies, crackers, pasta and bread.

If you prefer to eat organically, change the search to "organic markets" instead of "supermarkets."

How to Find Restaurants with Gluten-Free Menus

This time replace "supermarkets" with "gluten-free." "Gluten-free Coronado Island" should bring up local restaurants that offer a gluten-free menu.

Again, you'll want to note the name, phone number, and location of the places that sound interesting. You might find reviews from people who have eaten at these particular restaurants, which will help you decide if you want to eat there.

How to Find a Room with a Kitchen

The search for a room with a kitchen can be difficult. Sometimes they don't exist or are not affordable. It will cost more, but you'll save money in the long run by eating in. Plus, the amenities of a kitchen make it possible to have a relaxing, worry-free vacation.

Enter the search term "Coronado Island suites," which should bring up some hotels or motels with kitchens. Several major chains have affordable suites as they've recognized the need for travelers to feel like they're in a warm, homey, comfortable environment, especially if they stay for a long period of time.

Alternatively, you might look for a short-term rental condo or home. You can find daily and weekly rates on websites like Vacation Rental By Owner at www.vrbo.com.

Why Do You Need a Kitchen?

The hardest gluten-free meal to eat when traveling is breakfast. Having a kitchen is wonderful. Most continental breakfasts served by hotels consist mainly of toast, cereal and pastries. Hot items such as eggs and bacon are often served buffet style, and are red flags for cross-contamination.

But with a kitchen, you can make your own breakfast. And after you eat, you can go out for a nice coffee or tea.

Lunch can also be a tricky meal. And then there's snacking, especially if you have kids. With a kitchen, you will be able to keep them happy, healthy and gluten-free much more easily.

A quality kitchen should be equipped with a refrigerator, stove and microwave. Having them at your disposal will make it easy to take gluten-free restaurant leftovers back to your room.

But will you have to buy everything at the supermarket to stock your kitchen? What if the local supermarket doesn't carry your favorite gluten-free crackers? One thing I've learned is that you should pack a lot of gluten-free food and bring it with you – even if you're flying.

What to Pack

Can you travel with gluten-free food? Of course you can! My family and I have been known to fill an entire suitcase with gluten-free food.

So what would be good to pack? Non-perishable gluten-free items in air-tight containers, such as:
- Boxed cereal
- Pre-packaged meals like those from Go Picnic
- Pamela's flour mix (for making pancakes)
- Bread
- Crackers
- Cookies

- Soup
- Small bags of spices to season your meals (this is a good one!)
- Protein bars

Being equipped with gluten-free food will save money, and will be a lifesaver if you end up arriving in the middle of the night thanks to travel delays.

Now, get ready for one of the most challenging parts of traveling: Finding gluten-free food in an airport.

How to Eat Gluten-Free in an Airport

The only thing more difficult than getting through airport security is finding gluten-free food.

As opposed to franchises like Applebee's or Chili's that now offer gluten-free meals, few airports in the United States have restaurants that cater to gluten-free clientele. None of the options will be ideal, so you might end up eating junk food if your flight gets delayed.

As a back-up, have a list handy of gluten-free candy bars to buy at the newsstand along with a bottle of water. Remember, you can bring packaged food into the airport and through security, but you can't take liquids through. Check with the Transportation Security Administration about what you can bring (most airlines offer this information on their websites).

Pack things like dried jerky, crackers, chips, dried fruit and nuts in your carry-on luggage as traveling can be very unpredictable. You never know when they might come in handy.

Another idea is to pack and eat a gluten-free lunch at the airport. Come into the airport, check your bags, find a place to sit and eat your bagged lunch, then go through security.

If you have a layover, check the in-airport restaurants to see if they have anything gluten-free. If nothing is available you can always get a cup of fruit, which is great because flying can be dehydrating.

Don't forget the ice cream shops. It may be indulgent, but it's a much better choice than eating food containing gluten. Having jet lag is one thing; having jet lag and an upset system is another.

If you can't find anything in any of the shops or restaurants, get out your list of gluten-free candy bars and head to the newsstand.

Summary

- Find out what grocery stores carry gluten-free food at your destination.
- Find out what restaurants have gluten-free menus.
- Find a place with a kitchen that's close to stores where you can buy gluten-free food.
- Pack your favorite non-perishable gluten-free food.

- Be careful at airports since they tend to have few – if any – gluten-free options.
- Bring a pre-prepared meal to eat when you arrive at the airport before going through security.
- Have a list of chips and candy bars handy so you can buy snacks in the concourse.

Traveling can be stressful, but you can make your trip more relaxing by researching your options ahead of time. Making sure you have everything you need when you arrive at your destination will make you and your family happy campers!

Bon voyage!

Chapter 8: Reading Ingredient Lists

Gluten is a sneaky protein that is in a lot of different foods and products. Relatively few products tell you they are gluten-free right on the package. And for most products, it is unclear whether gluten is an ingredient or not.

So how can you find out if it's in your food?

Unfortunately, you will have to figure it out on your own. The best approach is to read the list of ingredients on the product. Reading ingredients can be a daunting task because some foods contain chemicals and ingredients you may have never heard of.

With practice and the right information, you'll be able to quickly find out if gluten is an ingredient.

How to Identify Gluten in an Ingredient List

Reading an ingredient list is one of the surest ways to tell if a product contains gluten. In this section I will show you how to read ingredient labels. From the ingredients you will be able to decide whether a food is safe, not safe, or does not give you enough information to decide.

If you are not sure about something, or it is not clear if there is gluten in the ingredients, then avoid the food or product. Just put it back on the shelf and go for something else. Easy as that!

"If you don't know, don't eat it!"

Gluten is never listed as an ingredient; therefore, you have to look for specific ingredients that contain gluten. Remembering all the ingredients that contain gluten makes label-reading complicated.

The good news is you won't need to check ingredients on a food every time you buy it. Generally speaking, food that is gluten-free today will still be that way next week. However, I recommend doing periodic ingredient checks on food you eat just to be sure. Although it is not the norm, ingredients sometimes change.

I have included a complete list of ingredients at the back of this book for your convenience. The list of ingredients will make it easy for you to check ingredients for gluten. If you would like a free copy of our Gluten-Free Ingredient List book, simply visit: http://happyglutenfree.com/ingredient-reference.

Now I will show you some sample ingredient labels and how to tell if a product is safe. It will take a while to learn how to read a label to see if the item is gluten-free. But remember, practice makes perfect. Every time you read ingredients you will get a little better at it.

Labelling Regulations

The Federal Nutrition Labeling and Education Act (NLEA) of 1990 require most food to bear nutrition labels and prescribe their form and content. They must state, among other things, the number of calories per serving and the amounts of fat, cholesterol, sodium, and fiber. Food that does not comply is deemed misbranded and invokes Food, Drug and Cosmetic Act (FD&CA) enforcement provisions.

The Food Allergen Labeling and Consumer Protection Act (FALCPA) of 2004 further amended the FD&CA. It requires food labels to state the presence of the eight major food allergens identified by the act. They are milk, eggs, fish, shellfish, tree nuts, wheat, peanuts, and soybeans. These eight allergens are responsible for 90% of all food allergies. Notice that barley, rye, and oats are not in the list of eight nor are any of wheat's many grain cousins like semolina, kamut, or triticale.

By law ingredients must be on most manufactured and processed food labels. However, some products and produce (i.e., at farmer's markets or organic outlets) don't have ingredient labels as they are not bound by the same food labeling laws. In that case, you should consult the manufacturer or producer about the ingredients and possible gluten contamination.

Reading a Label

Imagine you're at the grocery store and you've picked up a product you are interested in. Usually on the side of the box or back of package is a typical ingredient list that looks like the ones in Figures 1-4 below.

Note: In each of the images below, I put red box lines around the ingredient(s) that either contain gluten or could potentially be a gluten ingredient.

Ingredients: MARBLED COLBY AND MONTEREY JACK
CHEESES (PASTEURIZED MILK, CHEESE CULTURE, SALT,
ENZYMES, ANNATTO [COLOR]), NATAMYCIN (A
NATURAL MOLD INHIBITOR), BAKED WHOLE WHEAT
CRACKERS (WHOLE WHEAT, SOYBEAN OIL, SALT,
MONOGLYCERIDES).

Figure 1

The ingredient label in Figure 1 shows that wheat
is one of the ingredients. You would want to avoid
this product. The example in Figure 1 is a cheese and
crackers "to go" product. Any prepackaged food with
crackers likely contains gluten unless it specifies
"gluten-free" on the box or package.

The next example is not so obvious. It is a candy
bar that has barley malt in the ingredients. Barley malt
is an ingredient that contains gluten:

Ingredient Declaration:

MILK CHOCOLATE (SUGAR, COCOA BUTTER, SKIM MILK, CHOCOLATE, LACTOSE, MILKFAT, SOY LECITHIN, ARTIFICIAL FLAVOR), CORN SYRUP, SUGAR, HYDROGENATED PALM KERNEL OIL AND/OR PALM OIL, SKIM MILK, LESS THAN 2% - MILKFAT, COCOA POWDER PROCESSED WITH ALKALI, MALTED BARLEY, LACTOSE, SALT, EGG WHITES, CHOCOLATE, ARTIFICIAL FLAVOR.

Figure 2

The ingredient label in Figure 3 is not so clear. It turns out that the food is gluten-free, but it was not obvious from reading the ingredients. I had to contact the manufacturer and they informed me that there are no gluten ingredients:

INGREDIENTS:
CORN SYRUP, SUGAR, HYDROGENATED PALM KERNEL OIL AND/OR PALM OIL, FRUIT JUICE FROM CONCENTRATE (APPLE, STRAWBERRY, LEMON, ORANGE, CHERRY), LESS THAN 2% - CITRIC ACID, DEXTRIN GELATIN, FOOD STARCH-MODIFIED, NATURAL AND ARTIFICIAL FLAVORS, ASCORBIC ACID (VITAMIN C), COLORING (RED 40, YELLOW 6, YELLOW 5, BLUE 1).

Figure 3

Vague ingredients like 'Natural' or 'Artificial Flavors' are the most frustrating. Both terms are generalized and can contain gluten. Natural or artificial flavors can come from or contain barley. Many manufacturers I have spoken with note that they will list barley separately as an ingredient if it is used in the flavorings. Nonetheless, I still recommend contacting the manufacturer of any food you are not sure of.

Finally, this last ingredient list points out another important piece of information. Even if a product contains no gluten ingredients, you need to be informed about the facility and equipment where the product is made:

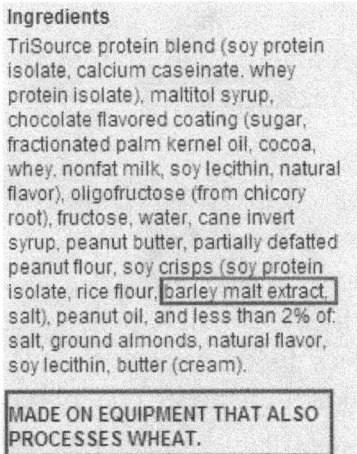

Ingredients
TriSource protein blend (soy protein isolate, calcium caseinate, whey protein isolate), maltitol syrup, chocolate flavored coating (sugar, fractionated palm kernel oil, cocoa, whey, nonfat milk, soy lecithin, natural flavor), oligofructose (from chicory root), fructose, water, cane invert syrup, peanut butter, partially defatted peanut flour, soy crisps (soy protein isolate, rice flour, barley malt extract, salt), peanut oil, and less than 2% of: salt, ground almonds, natural flavor, soy lecithin, butter (cream).

MADE ON EQUIPMENT THAT ALSO PROCESSES WHEAT.

Figure 4

The product label in Figure 4 contains barley malt extract which contains gluten. But also note the statement at the bottom of the label: "MADE ON EQUIPMENT THAT ALSO PROCESSES WHEAT." A similar statement you might see on labels is "MADE IN A FACILITY THAT ALSO PROCESSES WHEAT."

Products processed on or in equipment that also process wheat have a high risk of being contaminated with gluten, even if they don't contain any gluten ingredients.

Whether the food is manufactured on equipment or in a facility that contains wheat, it is worth talking with the manufacturer to find out more information. In some cases, manufacturers thoroughly clean their equipment between running every batch of food. In a case where the equipment is cleaned, you are probably safe.

If the manufacturer processes wheat on the same equipment but if the equipment is not sanitized, the risk of gluten contamination is too high and you should avoid the product.

Summary

Now you know how to check if a food is gluten-free. Reference the unsafe ingredient list at the end of this book to check foods as you review them. And remember, it takes practice to get good at reading labels. Don't worry if you have to spend a lot of time on it at first. You will get better!

Do you have to read every label in a supermarket to find out if products are gluten-free? Absolutely not, as I've done at lot of the legwork for you.

Next I'll talk about what food is gluten-free and safe to eat.

Chapter 9: Safe Gluten-Free Foods List

In this chapter, I will go over several foods that are gluten-free and safe to eat.

Shopping for gluten-free foods can be overwhelming and confusing. How do you know what foods are safe to eat? I talked about how to read ingredient labels so you can identify gluten-free foods. But that will take forever, won't it?

It does take time to figure out your own personal list of gluten-free foods that you like and that are available at supermarkets in your area. To help you along I have put together a list of several

In addition to giving you tips on what to look for, I'll provide names of several widely available gluten-free products you can shop for today.

Gluten-Free Food You Can Buy Today

I've divided gluten-free food into categories and brands you can find in most grocery stores. Depending on where you live and the size of your town, some of these may not be available (I've also listed websites where you can buy food online later in the chapter). But produce like fruits and vegetables, dairy and meat are available everywhere.

Produce

You can choose whatever fruits and vegetables you want from the produce section. Although some markets may have wheat grass available, you should avoid it. Otherwise, you can have your choice from what is available.

You already know about the benefits of eating fresh produce. However, it is worth noting that as you transition off gluten your body will need water and nutrients more than ever. What better way to give your body what it needs than with fresh fruits and vegetables?

Watch out for the dip that comes on a pre-made veggie tray (aka: crudités) may not be gluten-free. If you're in a hurry, grab a veggie tray and a bottle of salad dressing like Newman's Own Ranch Dressing for dipping your vegetables. Better yet, buy fresh vegetables, cut them up, organize them creatively on a tray, and put gluten-free ranch dressing in a bowl. Voila! Your tummy will appreciate the effort, and your guests won't know the difference.

Meat

Meat is an excellent source of protein and iron, which is especially important as your body heals. Avoid buying pre-marinated cuts of meat. Even if the meat doesn't contain gluten, marinades from unknown sources can cause havoc to your system.

You can make your own spice rubs and marinades. Single ingredient spices from McCormick's, Tone's, and Spice Islands are all gluten-free. Have fun and be inventive mixing different flavors together.

Several deli meats are gluten-free. But be cautious about ordering sliced meats (or cheeses) at the deli counter. The slicers and counters may be cross-contaminated with gluten from other products!

To that end, pre-packaged deli meat is the safest way to go. Although these brands make gluten-free deli meat, check the label to be sure:

- Hormel Natural Choice Meats
- Boar's Head
- Buddig
- Oscar Mayer

Since gluten can be used as an ingredient to add flavor and texture, other types of meat products to watch out for are chorizo, sausage, hot dogs, and "loaf" products like olive loaf.

These are some brands that are safe to eat:
- Coleman Naturals Hot Dogs
- Boulder Sausage (their sausage varieties are labeled gluten-free on the package)
- Johnsonville Ground Sausage
- Smithfield Smoked Sausage Loops
- Hillshire Farms Smoked Bratwurst
- Wellshire Farms Original Deli Franks
- Ball Park Singles Beef Franks

It may seem obvious, but you should avoid beer bratwurst since beer contains gluten. You can make your own at home with a gluten-free beer brand like Bards.

Bread

Gluten-free breads are typically found in the freezer section with the "organic foods". Gluten-free baked goods don't sell quickly since there is a limited amount of consumers who eat it. And they tend to have fewer preservatives, so it is more economical for stores to keep them frozen.

You may have to shop for gluten-free bread at a Whole Foods or other natural food stores if your supermarket doesn't carry them. Some bakeries are now carrying gluten-free bread, but you should ask about cross-contamination (i.e., do they have separate counters and containers to cook the bread in?) before you buy.

The best gluten-free breads are from:
- Rudy's Gluten-Free Bakery
- Udi's Gluten-Free Bakery
- Canyon Bakehouse

All three brands are distributed nationally.
Note: Rudy's and Udi's both make regular breads too – so be sure you are buying the gluten-free variety.

Gluten-free bread can be expensive, so expect to pay $5.00 or more per loaf (you can often find online coupons on the company's website).

Alternatively, to save money you can make good gluten-free bread from scratch or by using a bread machine. It's only marginally less expensive but the smell of bread baking in your kitchen and the fresh, homemade taste is well worth the effort.

Pasta

Pasta is a staple in most households. But are there tolerable gluten-free options are available?

Yes!

The best gluten-free pasta is made from brown rice flour, and is comparable to wheat-based pasta in taste and texture. Gluten-free pasta releases more starch than traditional pasta, so they should be rinsed well in the colander after cooking. Always cook your gluten-free pasta al dente; otherwise it will be mushy and sticky.

Gluten-free pasta may be located with regular pastas, or it may be in the natural food aisle. Many stores now have gluten-free designated areas, so check with a stock person if you can't find it.

The brands I like best are:
- Tinkyada Rice Pasta
- DeBoles
- Annie's Homegrown

Tinkyada and DeBoles make all types of pasta including spaghetti, macaroni, penne, spirals and others. Tinkyada also make lasagna noodles. DeBoles and Annie's both make a gluten-free macaroni and cheese.

Annie's and DeBoles also make wheat pasta. So be sure the package you buy states the pasta is gluten-free.

Flour

I am listing flour here because you will find baking to be the most economical way to enjoy things like pancakes, cookies, muffins, and bread. In general, baking with gluten-free flour is harder than baking with regular flour. But not all foods are more difficult to bake. For example, pancakes are easy to make gluten-free as are good chocolate chip cookies – if you have the right flour on hand.

You will find several different gluten-free flours available. Each one uses a unique blend of individual gluten-free grain flours. Brown rice flour and white rice flour are the most popular ingredients in gluten-free flour mixes as are tapioca starch and sorghum flour.

Contrary to what labels on many gluten-free flour mixes say, they don't make easy "one-for-one" replacements for wheat flour as they taste different and give food a different texture. Taking a recipe that uses wheat flour and trying to substitute gluten-free flour can result in disappointment, especially if you're new to using it. But there are wonderful, tasty exceptions.

You get the best results by using recipes that are tailored to being made gluten-free. I encourage you to experiment and see what works best for your taste.

Following are what I consider the best pre-made gluten-free flour mixes and what they work best for. They are relatively easy to find in stores and online:

- Pamela's Gluten-Free Pancake Mix (pancakes, crepes, cookies)
- Bob's Red Mill Gluten-Free Flour (easiest to find, best for cookies)
- Bisquick Gluten-Free Flour (great for muffins)
- Betty Crocker Gluten-Free Cake Mix (chocolate or vanilla)
- Betty Crocker Gluten-Free Brownie Mix

I use Pamela's mix every weekend to make pancakes, and my family loves it. The Betty Crocker mixes are located with the cake mixes, and say "gluten-free" right on the box.

You may also see several individually packaged gluten-free flours at your store. These are generally from Bob's Red Mill but other brands offer them too. These are flours you will need as you get into making your own flour mixes. Legendary gluten-free cooks like Bette Hagman and Carol Fenster have flour combination recipes tailored to baking various kinds of bread and cake.

Dairy

If you can tolerate milk products, you'll be thrilled to know that many dairy items are gluten-free. However, people newly diagnosed with celiac disease are often lactose-intolerant, so they have to avoid consuming dairy until their bodies are healed.

If you can tolerate dairy, these are foods you can safely eat:

Eggs

- Eggs (if cooking eggless – such as with Ener-G powder or Egg Beaters -- make sure it's gluten-free)

Milk

- Half-and-Half, whipping cream, skim, 1%, 2%, and whole milk are all safe to drink.

However, not all flavored or non-dairy milks are gluten-free. So it is best to check the ingredients before you buy.

There some milk varieties that are gluten-free:

- Nesquik, all ready-to-drink flavors
- Coffee-mate, all flavors
- Horizon, all flavors including chocolate and strawberry
- Organic Valley Eggnog and Soy Milk (vanilla)
- Buttermilk
- Pacific Natural Foods Almond, Hazelnut, Rice, and Soy Milk

Cheese

Is cheese gluten-free? Most of it is, but not all. For example, blocks of cheddar, Monterey Jack, and Swiss are safe. Bags of pre-shredded Kraft mozzarella, cheddar, or Parmesan are fine.

These are some other safe cheeses:

- Kraft Singles
- Laughing Cow Babybel and Wedges
- Frigo Ricottas
- Athenos cheeses
- Sargento shredded and sliced varieties
- Velveeta Regular
- Tillamook cheeses

Sour Cream and Yogurt

Sour cream and yogurt are two dairy products you'll probably have on hand on a regular basis. Here are a few gluten-free national brands:

- Daisy Sour Cream
- Knudsen Sour Cream and Yogurt
- Stonyfield Fat Free, Low Fat and Whole Milk Yogurt
- Tillamook Sour Cream and Yogurt
- Yoplait yogurts specify if they are gluten-free on the package

Cereal

It's nice to have a few boxes of cereal on hand, because it makes an easy breakfast or snack:

- General Mills Chocolate, Cinnamon, Corn, Honey Nut and Rice Chex
- Eco-Planet Original Instant Hot Cereal
- Nature's Path Amazon Frosted Flakes or Koala Crisp

Don't assume that all General Mills Chex cereal is gluten-free. Look for "gluten-free" on the front of the box. Nature's Path gluten-free cereals taste good, and they make several that are fun for kids.

Pasta Sauces

Pasta sauce is obviously great on pasta. But you can also use marinara as a pizza sauce or dip for gluten-free bread sticks. I've used Newman's Own Marinara for pizza sauce and dipping for years.

Unfortunately, not all pasta sauces are gluten-free. But these sauces currently are:

- Dei Fratelli
- Classico red and white sauces
- Newman's Own

Salad Dressings

Like pasta sauce, salad dressing can be used for more than just salad. It can also be used as a dip or marinade. Here are some gluten-free salad dressing options:

- Bolthouse Farms
- Cookwell & Company Cracked Black Pepper Vinaigrette
- Newman's Own Ranch, Balsamic Vinaigrette, and Caesar
- Kraft Thousand Island and Ranch

Not all salad dressings are gluten-free. So read the ingredients (you're probably getting good at that by now!), and check with the manufacturer to be sure what is and is not safe.

Summary

Several foods that you are familiar with are gluten-free. On top of that, meat, produce, and many dairy products are safe for you to eat and they are available everywhere.

Some products are more specialized and hard to find. In that case, I recommend searching for the products on either of these websites:

Amazon.com: In addition, you get free two-day shipping and cheap overnight shipping with an Amazon Prime membership.

Celiac.com - The Gluten-Free Mall: Is one of the original online gluten-free supermarkets.

You have many gluten-free food options available. But you should also be aware of the foods to avoid. I will talk about those in the next chapter.

Chapter 10: Foods to Avoid

You're probably realizing by now that eating gluten-free is very possible. You may recognize many of the brands listed above, and may have even used them before.

The food I discussed above is safe, but what about food that isn't? There are three categories of food in every grocery store: Safe, unsafe, and those you're unsure of.

As I discussed earlier, gluten hides in many places. By understanding what food contains gluten, you will be aware of what foods to stay away from.

Why should you learn about what food is unsafe?

Some products, like Wheaties, obviously have gluten as an ingredient. But with others, it is not so obvious. Like Soy Sauce, for example (which is made from fermented wheat). Or Play-Doh, which is a product made with wheat flour. Knowing what foods are safe is critical but it is also important to be familiar with food to avoid when you eat a gluten-free diet.

Food to Avoid When Eating Gluten-Free

The primary grains that contain gluten are wheat, barley, and rye. But did you know there are several wheat and barley-related grains you should also avoid?

- Spelt
- Kamut
- Club
- Durum
- Bulgur
- Einkorn
- Semolina
- Graham

A friend of a friend once asked if I wanted several kinds of unused gluten-free flour. They had tried going gluten-free since they had related symptoms. For some reason eating gluten-free had not helped them. So now they were getting rid of these flours and I said I would take them. Well, one of the bags they gave us was semolina flour (which is not gluten-free). Yikes!

No wonder they weren't getting better, as they had not truly eliminated gluten from their diet! This is sad, because they never gave their body the chance to become fully healed from consuming a healthy, gluten-free diet.

What Food is Made With Gluten?

To begin feeling your best, and to become symptom-free, you need to completely eliminate gluten from your diet, which of course means eliminating food that contains gluten.

So what kinds of common food are made with gluten?

- Bread
- Pasta
- Crusts
- Muffins
- Cookies
- Cake
- Cupcakes
- Croutons
- Flour tortillas
- Tarts
- Bagels
- Buns
- Cereal
- Donuts
- Green chili
- Gravy
- Pudding
- Breading
- Bullion
- Soup

- Malted milkshake
- Pizza
- Nutrition bars
- Fried food (including French fries)
- Enchilada, Hoisin and teriyaki sauces

These basic food items make up hundreds of the most popular meals in today's culture. No wonder going gluten-free can be so hard at first!

Were you surprised by any of the ingredients on that list? I myself was shocked to learn about all the places where gluten hides.

Where Else Does Gluten Hide?

I talked earlier about the characteristics of gluten that make it so useful. Following are other non-food products that may contain gluten, such as:
- Shampoo
- Conditioner
- Cosmetics
- Lipstick
- Makeup
- Lip balm
- Sun block
- Medicine
- Play-Doh
- Kid's paints

If you have children note that Play-Doh is made with wheat flour, so it is one to watch out for because kids like to eat it! The Kaplan Early Learning Company offers a gluten-free alternative to Play-Doh for sale on Amazon.com. I have included a recipe to make your own version in the "Recipes" which is located at the back of this book.

Summary

Some surprising foods and products contain gluten. By understanding what those foods and products are, you know what foods to stay away from.

Now that you know about food that is gluten-free and safe and food that's unsafe, you might be wondering how you can you eat gluten-free without blowing your food budget. My next chapter, "Be Thrifty," gives tips on how to eat healthy while saving money.

Chapter 11: Eating Gluten-Free on a Budget

It is a fact that eating gluten-free is expensive. So how do you keep costs low and your spirits high? The key is to focus your budget on inexpensive food that does the best job of satisfying your family's hunger and your dietary needs.

The food industry has people hooked on eating cheap, easily accessible, throw-away products. Ever witness how fast a bag of Oreo's cookies disappears from the pantry? You might not know it yet, but the gluten-free equivalent of Oreo's costs almost double (did you hear your wallet scream?).

You don't have money to waste. So why spend it on sugary gluten-free food that provides little to no nutritional value?

Why is Gluten-Free Food More Expensive?

Before going gluten-free you were probably used to buying bread and cookies at reasonably low prices. But now that you are on a new diet, gluten-free equivalents are produced in smaller batches. And the ingredients to make those equivalents – like gluten-free flour -- are more expensive.

Additionally, some gluten-free food manufacturers use special tests to certify that they comply with gluten-free requirements -- an expense that ultimately gets passed on to you. It's simple economics that higher production costs result in higher food prices. Hopefully, as more people eat gluten-free, more gluten-free food will be produced and the cost will come down.

What Gluten-Free Food is the Most Expensive?

The most expensive gluten-free foods are those that use specialty gluten-free ingredients. For example, a small bag half-pound bag of gluten-free brown rice flour, which is a common ingredient in baked goods, costs about the same as a two pound bag of wheat flour.

What does that tell you? If that bag of brown rice flour is expensive for you, it is expensive for the manufacturer too.

It makes sense then, that the most expensive gluten-free foods are baked goods that use expensive ingredients. Foods like cookies, cakes, cupcakes, breads, muffins, and nutrition bars are the most expensive.

You might say, "Well, it's baked in a dedicated gluten-free facility. And that's supposed to be a good thing." Well, yes it is. But you're paying extra for that manufacturing safety. There are healthy gluten-free food items that cost the same no matter what diet you're on. So you need to find the ones that are healthy and less expensive.

What Gluten-Free Food is Less Expensive?

Produce. Fruits and vegetables are naturally gluten-free and they satisfy hunger and nutritional needs.

- Meat, as long as it's not pre-seasoned, pre-marinated, or full of flavor enhancers
- Many plain dairy products
- Many chips and crackers are gluten-free
- Nuts

None of these require special ingredients or handling to make sure they are gluten-free. They naturally come that way.

You may be thinking you will never get your family to eat fruits and vegetables. And that you can't live without sandwiches and buns (remember the gluten-free alternatives I mentioned previously).

It is a challenge to keep everyone happy at mealtime. But you only have so much money to spend on food. So what can you serve on a tight budget?

How to Keep Costs Down

If you're on a tight budget the number one priority should be feeding your family healthy, nutritional food.

Staples

- Fruits (great for breakfast or a snack), vegetables, nuts and meat provide the highest protein and nutritional value.
- Salad makes a great meal by itself, or as a side for any meal.
- Dairy is second in cost efficiency: Eggs and cheese are as important as milk (you can always buy dry milk, and it's less expensive than fresh).
- Next in importance is cereal (again, several General Mills Chex cereals are gluten-free. They're the most cost-effective and

nutritional since they're fortified with vitamins and minerals).

- Gluten-free pasta and bread. Avoid buying gluten-free buns as they can be pricey. It won't take your family long to get used to eating hot dogs and hamburgers without them, which can save you a ton of money every year.

Snacks
- You can buy large inexpensive bags of gluten-free potato or corn chips.
- Nuts can be expensive, but they fill you up fast so you need to consume less.
- You can buy big boxes of gluten-free Crunchmaster Multi-Grain Crackers at places like Costco or Sam's Club.

Beverages
If your family likes sweet beverages, opt for frozen concentrates instead of sodas or bottled juice.

You may have noticed that I haven't mentioned cookies, muffins or ice cream. If you have money left over for such treats, that's great. But if you're working with a tight budget, focus on the food that will sustain you and your pocketbook!

Summary

- Gluten-free food is more expensive because it costs more to make.
- Gluten-free bread, cupcakes, cakes, muffins, and cookies are the most expensive.
- Produce, meat, plain dairy products and chips are less expensive.
- Buying protein-rich and nutritional food will keep your family well-fed and your budget in check.

Eating gluten-free is a balancing act between enjoyable yet affordable food. Things like cookies, cakes and muffins are so yummy that it can seem like a sacrifice to give them up.

But you have to keep your family healthy, so focus your budget on protein-rich, high nutrient gluten-free food such as meat, fruits and vegetables.

Conclusion

My primary goal in writing *Gluten-Free for Beginners* was to help you overcome obstacles to becoming gluten-free. It takes a lot of devotion to make a transition like this to your diet, so I applaud you for making the effort.

After studying this book...
- You are well-armed to lead a healthy gluten-free life.
- You know what gluten is, and how it can negatively affect you and your family.
- You know how to make your home safely gluten-free, and that should feel really, really good.
- You have learned that cross-contamination is too critical to ignore. And now that you're aware of it you'll be much less likely to accidentally eat gluten.
- You know what steps to take to find a good gluten-free meal while traveling or at restaurants.
- You have learned how to form a gluten-free diet plan and communicate your needs to people such as family members and wait staff who come in contact with your food.
- You have learned that not all food is clearly labeled gluten-free, but that doesn't mean

you can't eat them. With a little research you can find out if it's safe for consumption.

A Friendly Request

I hope you have enjoyed reading this book and that you learned some helpful information from it.

Positive reviews from people like you are extremely important to me. If you have benefited from reading it would you please leave a review?

If I need to fix anything in this book please let me know. Any typos, any ideas to improve, please let me know so I can improve this book.

It is important to me to make high quality products. So this means, if you find something I have overlooked then I want to hear about it.

Send your feedback to my email address: jim@happyglutenfree.com. This email will come directly to me – not an assistant or other gatekeeper.

Thank you in advance for your review!

Other Books By James L. Shirley

Check out these other helpful books
Gluten-Free Diet: A Shopping Guide

10 Tasty Taco Recipes

Restaurant Questions

Below are some good questions to ask (feel free to add any particular questions relating to your special needs):

1. What gluten-free menu items do they have?
2. What precautions do they take to keep food gluten-free?
3. If they serve pancakes or hamburgers, are the gluten-free ones cooked on the same griddle as the non-gluten?
4. Is the salad pre-mixed with croutons or other gluten-containing toppings?
5. Ask if you can be seated with a gluten-knowledgeable member of the wait staff as some servers are more aware than others.

Keep in mind that researching which restaurants serve gluten-free food only needs to be done periodically. It's a good idea to check every six months or so to see what changes have occurred -- and any time there is a change in management -- to ensure the same protocols for gluten-free dining are being followed.

But even if you know the restaurant has a gluten-free menu, you should talk with your server upon arrival to make sure they handle your order properly. Always communicate to your wait person that you have to eat gluten-free. This is an outline of steps to follow when you arrive:

1. Ask for the gluten-free menu before being seated.
2. When your server comes to take your drink order, let them know you intend to order from the gluten-free menu.
3. Ask if they can recommend any gluten-free appetizers. This is a great way to alert them that you'll be eating gluten-free throughout the meal.
4. Ask which salad dressings are gluten-free (don't be surprised if they don't know as this usually isn't a topic of discussion in the kitchen). Places like Amazon.com sells gluten-free salad dressings in portable packets. It's a good idea to keep some in your car or handbag in case a restaurant can't tell you if its dressings are gluten-free.
5. Confirm that your salad isn't pre-mixed with croutons or any toppings containing gluten.

Your meal should go well if the answers to all your questions have been answered to your satisfaction.

Recipes

The next several pages contain recipes for fun dough, breakfast, lunch, and dinner. These recipes go along with the menu recommendations from earlier in the book.

Kids Fun Dough Recipe

Make your own Play-Doh type dough. (Recipe from Parents Magazine)

   1/2 cup rice flour
   1/2 cup corn starch
   1/2 cup salt
   2 teaspoons cream of tartar (that'll keep the kids from eating it!)
   1 cup water
   1 teaspoon cooking oil

Mix the ingredients. At this point, you can add food coloring for fun. Cook and stir on low heat for 3 minutes or until a ball is formed. Cool completely and then store in a seal-able plastic bag.

Breakfast Menu Recipes

Berry Smoothie

1 cup fresh or frozen berries, any kind
1/2 cup apple juice
1/2 cup milk
1/4 cup yogurt
1/2 teaspoon vanilla

Combine all the ingredients in a mixer and blend until smooth. Makes two servings.

Breakfast Pancakes

1 cup Pamela's Pancake Mix
3/4 cup milk or water
1 tablespoon olive oil
1/4 teaspoon vanilla
1 large egg

Mix the milk, egg, oil, and vanilla together well. Add the Pamela's mix in and stir until a lumpy batter forms. Cook the pancakes on a griddle at 325 degrees Fahrenheit. Makes four servings.

Breakfast Tacos

1 tablespoon butter
5 ounces chorizo (about 1/3 of a pound)
1/2 medium white onion, diced
1 jalapeño pepper, diced
5 large eggs

Also:

8 - 12 corn tortillas
grated Monterey Jack cheese
pico de gallo
1/4 teaspoon chili powder (optional)

Warm corn tortillas in aluminum foil at 300 degrees for 15 minutes.

Whisk the eggs in a medium bowl and set aside. Melt the butter in a large skillet over medium heat. Add the chorizo and break it into small chunks. Fry until the chorizo is browned and the fat has mostly cooked away. Add the onion and pepper. Let cook about two minutes before adding the egg. Mix with a spatula until the eggs are scrambled. Lightly sprinkle chili powder on the mixture for a spicy kick.

Remove the corn tortillas and stack two per taco on each plate. Spoon the chorizo egg mixture on each taco, cover with cheese, and garnish with pico de gallo.

Cheese Omelette

Non-stick cooking spray or 1 teaspoon butter
2 eggs
1/2 teaspoon salt
1/2 teaspoon black pepper
1/4 teaspoon dill
1/8 cup gluten-free, shredded cheddar cheese

Heat a small non-stick skillet over medium heat. Spray the skillet with the cooking spray or melt the butter.

In a small bowl, whisk the eggs and seasonings together. Pour the egg mixture into the skillet. Cook over medium heat, swirling the pan occasionally to ensure the eggs uniformly cover the bottom of the pan. Flip the omelet when it is almost set. Cook an additional 30 seconds. Sprinkle the cheese over one side, fold the omelet and slide it onto a plate. Makes one serving.

Lunch Menu Recipes

3 Cheese Pasta Bake

1 pound gluten-free penne
2 cups heavy cream
1 (14-ounce) can crushed tomatoes
2 cup bag shredded Italian cheese
1/2 teaspoon salt
1/2 teaspoon black pepper
1/2 teaspoon nutmeg
1/2 cup chopped fresh basil

Prepare the pasta according to package directions. Rinse and drain.

Preheat the oven to 400 degrees Fahrenheit. In a large bowl, combine the remaining ingredients. Stir in the pasta. Pour this mixture into a 9 by 13 inch pan. Bake for 20 minutes, or until the top is browned. Makes six servings.

Asian Coleslaw

Dressing:

>1/4 cup gluten-free Tamari soy sauce
>juice and zest of one lime
>1 teaspoon sugar
>1/2 teaspoon salt
>1/2 teaspoon black pepper
>1/2 teaspoon ginger
>1/2 teaspoon cayenne pepper
>1/2 teaspoon minced garlic
>1/2 cup vegetable oil

Salad:

>2 cups cabbage, sliced thinly
>1/2 cup chopped red pepper
>2 carrots, grated
>2 green onions, chopped
>1/4 cup cilantro, chopped
>1/4 cup chopped peanuts

Combine the dressing ingredients and refrigerate for up to four hours. Toss the dressing with the salad ingredients and refrigerate or serve immediately. Makes six servings.

Broccoli Cheese Soup

1/2 pound broccoli, washed and cut in 2 inch
pieces
2 cups milk
2 tablespoons cornstarch
1 cup shredded cheddar cheese
1/2 teaspoon salt
1/2 teaspoon onion powder
1/2 teaspoon black pepper
1/2 teaspoon nutmeg

Steam or boil the broccoli until tender. Puree in a
food processor or blender. Combine the broccoli with
the milk and cornstarch and heat over medium heat,
stirring frequently, until the mixture begins to thicken.
Add the remaining ingredients and cook an additional
5 minutes, or until the cheese melts. Makes six
servings.

Chicken and Spinach Salad

Dressing:

1/4 cup vinegar
1 tablespoon orange juice concentrate
1/2 teaspoon dry mustard powder
1/2 teaspoon salt
1/2 teaspoon black pepper

1 teaspoon honey
1/2 cup vegetable oil

Salad:

2 cups washed spinach
1/2 cup shredded chicken
1/2 cup chopped pecans
1 avocado, diced
1/2 cup gluten-free feta cheese
1 (8 ounce) can mandarin oranges, drained

Toss the salad ingredients in a large bowl. In a smaller bowl, combine the vinegar, orange juice, honey and seasonings. Slowly add the oil, whisking for 30 seconds, or until smooth. Refrigerate the dressing for at least one hour prior to serving for best flavor. Makes six servings.

Strawberry Salad

Dressing:

1/4 cup red wine vinegar
1/2 teaspoon dry mustard
1/2 teaspoon salt
1/2 teaspoon black pepper
2 tablespoons gluten-free strawberry jam
1 tablespoon diced onion
1/2 cup vegetable oil

Salad:

> 2 cups spinach or baby greens
> 1/2 cup sliced strawberries
> 1/2 cup slivered almonds
> 1/4 cup shelled edamame
> 1/4 cup diced red bell pepper
> 1/4 cup crumbed, gluten-free bacon

Combine all the dressing ingredients in a blender. Whirl for 30 seconds, or until thick and completely combined. Refrigerate for at least two hours to blend flavors. Toss with salad ingredients and serve immediately. Makes six servings.

Tomato Basil Pasta

2 Roma tomatoes, diced
1/2 cup fresh mozzarella, cut in 1 inch cubes
1/2 cup fresh, chopped basil
1/2 cup olive oil
1/2 teaspoon salt
1/2 teaspoon black pepper
1/2 teaspoon minced garlic
1 pound gluten-free penne pasta

Combine all the ingredients except the pasta in a large serving dish. Allow it to sit for 30 minutes to allow the flavors to meld. Boil the pasta according to package directions, rinse and drain. Toss the pasta with the tomato mixture and serve. Makes six servings.

Dinner Menu Recipes

Beef Burgundy

2 strips gluten-free bacon
1/2 cup diced onion
1/2 cup chopped mushrooms
1 pound stew meat or pot roast, cut in 2 inch cubes
1 cup red wine
1 cup gluten-free beef broth
2 tablespoons tapioca flour
2 tablespoons tomato paste
1/2 teaspoon salt
1/2 teaspoon black pepper
1/2 teaspoon minced garlic
1/2 teaspoon thyme

Cook the bacon in a large skillet until crispy and browned. Drain on paper towels and crumble. Add the onions and mushrooms to the bacon drippings and cook until tender, stirring frequently, 3 to 4 minutes. Place in the slow cooker. Brown the beef in the bacon drippings, until browned on all sides. Transfer to the slow cooker. Add the remaining ingredients, including the bacon, and cook on low 6 hours. Serve with mashed potatoes or gluten-free noodles. Makes six servings.

Note: Cornstarch is often used as a thickening agent in gluten-free cooking, but it breaks down with extended heat. Tapioca flour works better in the slow cooker. Makes six servings.

Chicken Cacciatore

2 tablespoons vegetable oil
4 boneless, skinless chicken breasts
1 onion, cut in rings
1 green bell pepper, cut in rings
1/2 cup mushrooms, sliced
1 clove garlic, minced
1 (14.5 ounce) can diced tomatoes, drained
1 (6 ounce) can tomato paste
1 cup water
1 teaspoon salt
1/2 teaspoon black pepper
1 teaspoon dried basil
1/2 teaspoon dried oregano

Heat the oil in a large skillet. Add the chicken breasts and sauté for 10 minutes, or until browned. Add the onions, peppers, and mushrooms and cook an additional 5 minutes. Stir in the remaining ingredients. Cover and simmer for 30 minutes. Makes six servings.

Chicken Enchiladas

1 tablespoon vegetable oil
1/4 cup minced onion
1 clove garlic, minced
1 (6 ounce) can diced green chiles
2 cups shredded chicken
1/2 teaspoon salt
1/2 teaspoon black pepper
1/2 teaspoon chipotle chili powder
1/2 teaspoon cumin
8 gluten-free corn tortillas
1/2 cup shredded cheddar or Mexican cheese

Enchilada Sauce:

2 cups gluten-free chicken broth
3 tablespoons chili powder
1/2 teaspoon garlic powder
1/2 teaspoon ground cumin
1/2 teaspoon chipotle chili powder
2 tablespoons cornstarch

Preheat the oven to 350 degrees Fahrenheit. To make the enchilada sauce, combine all the ingredients in a medium saucepan. Heat over medium high heat until the sauce boils and thickens, stirring frequently.

Heat the oil in a medium skillet. Add the onion and garlic and cook until tender. Add the remaining ingredients, except the corn tortillas and cheese and heat for 5 minutes, stirring to mix. Place the tortillas in a 9 by 13 inch baking dish and heat in the oven for 5 minutes to soften them. (cont'd)

To fill the tortillas, dip them in the enchilada sauce, lay them in the pan and fill each with ½ cup of the chicken and onion filling. Roll them up and place them, seam side down, in the pan. Top with the remaining enchilada sauce and the cheese. Bake for 30 minutes, or until bubbly. Makes six servings.

Grilled Salmon

3 tablespoons gluten-free Tamari soy sauce
juice and zest of one lemon
1 teaspoon minced garlic
1/2 teaspoon black pepper
1/2 teaspoon salt
4 salmon fillets

Combine the Tamari soy sauce, lemon juice and seasonings in a shallow dish or plastic bag. Place the salmon in the bag carefully and marinate for six hours or overnight. Drain. Heat the grill to medium high. Brush the grill grates with oil to prevent sticking. Grill the salmon 6 minutes on each side. Makes four servings.

Ground Beef Tacos

1 pound lean ground beef
1 cup red salsa
1 tablespoon garlic, minced (about 2 medium cloves)
1 1/2 teaspoons chili powder
1/2 teaspoon dried oregano
1/8 teaspoon cayenne pepper (optional)

Also:

8 - 12 taco shells
grated cheddar or Monterey Jack cheese
shredded romaine lettuce
1 chopped tomato
sour cream
salsa

Place a rack in the middle of the oven and warm to 170 degrees. Sprinkle grated cheddar cheese in the taco shells before you put them in the oven. The melted cheese keeps the taco shells from breaking so easily.

In a large skillet, warm the salsa and garlic over medium heat. Add the ground beef and break it up until it is crumbly. Cook until the meat is browned, about 12 minutes. If there is still grease in the pan, drain it off to avoid greasy tacos. Add the chili powder, oregano, and cayenne (if you use it) and mix well.

Spoon the meat into taco shells and serve. Have lettuce, cheese, sour cream, tomato, and salsa ready for garnishing.

Meatloaf

1 tablespoon vegetable oil
1/2 cup chopped onion
1/2 cup chopped red bell pepper
1/2 cup gluten-free bacon crumbles
1 pound lean ground beef
1 cup gluten-free oatmeal
1 egg, beaten
1 teaspoon salt
1/2 teaspoon black pepper
1/2 teaspoon thyme
3 tablespoons gluten-free ketchup
1 teaspoon dry mustard powder
1/2 teaspoon brown sugar

Preheat the oven to 350 degrees Fahrenheit. Heat the oil in a medium skillet. Add the onion and bell pepper and cook until tender. Combine the onion, pepper, bacon, ground beef, oatmeal, egg and seasonings in a large bowl. Mix thoroughly and place in a loaf pan or 8 inch baking dish. Combine the ketchup, mustard and brown sugar in a small bowl. Pour over the ground beef and smooth with a spoon. Bake for 45 minutes, or until the meatloaf is fully cooked. Makes four servings.

Teriyaki Chicken

4 boneless skinless chicken breasts
1/4 cup gluten-free teriyaki sauce
1/2 teaspoon minced garlic
1 tablespoon honey
juice and zest of one orange

Place the chicken breasts in a slow cooker. Stir together the remaining ingredients and pour over the chicken. Cook on low for 4 to 6 hours, turning the chicken halfway through. Makes four servings.

Thanks for reading!